Fuck you cancer!
Not with me!

3 Diagnoses 3 Fights 3 Victories

Acknowledgement

Special thanks goes to all the doctors, nurses and specialists who have accompanied me during these years.

To my friends and acquaintances who stood by me and cared for me. Especially my neighbor, who went shopping for me, a friend in Traunstein and friends in Erding, who raised me up and always had an open ear for me when I was mentally exhausted.

The thanks goes to the people who were there for me and helped me to cope with this heavy blow of fate and to fight against a cancer that should have killed me.

Table of contents

FOREWORD 7

2015 - THE NIGHTMARE BEGINS 9

DIAGNOSIS 9
THERAPY 10
GEHT´S ALSO ALTERNATIVE? 11

2018 - AND IT GOES ON 16

2019 - WON THE FIGHT? 23

WHAT NUTRITION HAS TO DO WITH CANCER 28

RECIPES AT A GLANCE: 31

MAGNESIUM CHLORIDE SOLUTION 31
LEMON CIDER VINEGAR DRINK.....................................33
SODIUM SOLUTION 34
.... 34
NUTRITIONAL SUPPLEMENTS 35

FURTHER TITLES OF THE AUTHOR 36

Foreword

"Anyone who eats a healthy diet, does a lot of sports and leads a balanced life will stay healthy and have a long life.“

In this or a similar way, society suggests to us that we do not need to be afraid of serious illnesses if we pay attention to our self and our body.

I've always looked out for myself. I did a lot of sports and had a healthy diet. My life was balanced, I was happy and had a great girlfriend who has been with me for many years.

Still got me. When I was diagnosed with cancer in 2015, it literally tore the floor under my feet.
After the first shock had been overcome, a fighting spirit developed in me that I had never experienced before.
I wanted to defeat cancer. No matter what it takes.

In this book, you read my story. How I got the diagnosis. About how my partner had left me because she couldn't or didn't want to see me die. And about how I finally defeated three different cancers in four years.

If you yourself are affected, I cannot guarantee that my methods will work for you. No one can. Because every person, every disease, is different.

But I can encourage you to test alternative methods, get another opinion at the right moment and then, if necessary, trust doctors and follow your gut feeling.

2015 - The nightmare begins

When in April 2015 my back pain got worse and worse, I first suspected that I might have a herniated disc or something similar. But since I had always done a lot of sports, I just couldn't imagine it. After all, I was very active and had a healthy diet. My back had not caused me any major problems so far.

When a herniated disc was finally ruled out, the doctors were at a loss. No one had any idea where the ever-increasing pain might come from.

The doctors desperately looked for the cause of the pain. After I got stronger and stronger complaints, however, the doctor suggested that I have a colonoscopy done.

The Diagnosis

It was already September when I went to the endocrinologist and the recommended colonoscopy could be performed.

And then there was the shock: bowel cancer!

Everything that came then ran more or less like a bad movie in front of me.

I was referred to Landshut Oncology and from there admitted to hospital. When the port for chemotherapy was implanted in me, I slowly began to realize what was actually happening to me here.

A port is a catheter that is usually implanted just below the collarbone directly under the skin in a vein near the heart. It is hardly visible from the outside but makes the treatment much easier.

The port should give me all kinds of medications. Morphine, chemo and even blood tests could be done over it. This is gentle on the veins, as there is no need to prick each time.

The application for severe disability followed with 80 %. Despite the planned chemo and radiation, which were to start in mid-November, my chance of survival was less than 5 %, since the tumor was over 5 cm in size and the neighbouring tissue was already severely affected.

In principle, I was practically dead.

This diagnosis had already begun to change me internally. Even if you hadn't looked at it from the inside, I wasn't the same any more at that time. The pain and fear of a serious illness alone had opened the doors to depression.

The Therapy

When I was backing home, and had time to think about everything in peace, I realized that I had hardly really internalized anything of what was told to me. It was only clear to me that I was seriously ill, had an extremely aggressive cancer and hardly any chance of survival.

But according to the doctors I should do myself the martyrdom of a chemo and radiation despite the so small chance of survival?

After a lot of consideration, I decided shortly before the beginning of the treatment not to let myself be treated as planned.
If I was almost dead anyway, I could also calmly consider whether and, if so, how I should be treated.
It was the end of November.

I used the coming weeks to get different opinions from different doctors and to be advised in several clinics. I learned about alternative treatments and acquired extensive knowledge about the disease that could kill me. And while I was doing all these things, I still seemed perfectly normal to outsiders.

Is alternative a way?

At the end of January 2016 I decided to be treated in the Proton Clinic in Munich (rptc.de).
Compared to conventional X-ray irradiation, irradiation with protons is more gentle on the surrounding tissue. In addition, the tumor is treated more specifically and is therefore destroyed right down to its DNA.
The proton irradiation with simultaneous chemo lasted a total of seven weeks. During this time, I was hospitalized in the clinic in Munich.
At first, it seemed like I could take it all very well. But after two weeks, the symptoms began to get worse and worse. I was accompanied by pain, open parts of the body and a lot of blood loss. I could hardly eat anything my digestion

and the bowel movement went crazy. The irradiation sites were sore and painful.

And as if the physical complaints weren't bad enough already, my partner of many years left me as well. She didn't want to see me miserably vegging out.

So, I had to process beside the pain also still that my girlfriend ended the relationship. After she had lost her brother to cancer only a few years earlier at a very young age, she did not have the strength to stand by me.

The depression was now in full swing. But who could blame me? There are always stories about how people defeated cancer, but I also heard about those who didn't make it. In the circle of acquaintances people told me again and again completely unconsidered some stories of people who had to give up their lives after chemo. And that it wasn't particularly constructive is self-explanatory.

And then there were the accusations I made to myself because my girlfriend had left. Had I done something wrong? Was it really "only" due to my illness or had she been playing with the idea of leaving me for some time? I didn't know. All I knew was she was gone. And left me alone with all the mess I was in.

When I was finally released in March, I had already eaten soup for four weeks. Solid food was no longer possible. Every sip hurt and I was grateful for every small portion I didn't have to puke again.

The dose of morphine was so high that I slept up to 23 hours a day. But at least I was able to withstand the extremely strong pain to some extent.

Since I was no longer able to take care of myself, I had temporarily moved to a friend in Erding.

The recovery and healing of the open wounds caused by the irradiation progressed very slowly.

But despite the first psychological problems, I had developed a fighting spirit that gave me the strength every day to stand up and continue fighting.

I wanted to defeat cancer and show everyone that a chance of survival below 5% could be enough to win this seemingly unconquerable battle.

On the web I found recommendations that sodium bicarbonate can help defeat cancer. There are physicians who administer sodium bicarbonate together with maple syrup to wash out the cells near the tumor.

Since I had the cancer directly in the intestine, I could fall back on the oral solution. And that's what I did. From the end of March, I drank two glasses a day with 5 grams each of baking soda dissolved in 0.2 litres of lukewarm water, mixed with two teaspoons of organic maple syrup. There were no side effects, so I could try it without hesitation. More than not helping, the stuff couldn't do that in me.

At the beginning of June, we finally went to Passau for rehabilitation. I refueled slowly, my strength returned. But there I realized that I couldn't go back home to my old apartment.

So after rehab, I needed a new home. Since I was still in the rehabilitation clinic, finding an apartment was very difficult. In the end I ended up in the Vogtland, far away from my home in Erding and my friends in Bavaria.

But since I had no choice in my situation but to take what I could get, I yielded to fate, packed my things and moved.

It wasn't just the broken relationship. I had been on sick leave for several months, only received sick pay and didn't know when I had a job again or if I would ever be able to work again. In such a situation, having to search for accommodation does not really facilitate the search for suitable housing.

Now it was the middle of July and slowly, but surely, the desire grew in me to be able to work again.
But how would that work? I was pumped full of morphine all the way to the top and was now dependent on it.
I couldn't work like that. No reasonable employer would give me a job in my condition.
So only rehab helped. Since a proper withdrawal in a clinic would take too long for me, I locked myself in an empty room at the beginning of August and did the withdrawal on my own. Cold! Without any help! Without substitutes. No painkillers. After a week of cruel pain, I had survived the worst. My head was clear, I didn't need morphine to deal with life anymore. I was ready for my second life.

Finding a job wasn't that easy. In the end, however, I found one in a company where I had worked before. Life finally started again. I was overjoyed.
But after four weeks I was disillusioned: I was away from morphine, but the pain came back. And grew stronger and stronger. So strong, I had to stay home again. Until the end of January I was still sick and struggled painfully and laboriously back into life.

But this time without morphine. I really wanted to hold on, because the cold turkey shouldn't have been for nothing.

In February, finally, I started a new attempt. On the outside I seemed to blossom, but on the inside, I was still plagued by pain, which I tried to ignore.

However, as the follow-up checks got better and better and the pain slowly subsided, I was convinced that things were finally going uphill again.

Until February 2018...

2018 - And it goes on

I have tried to ignore the pain that is now getting stronger again. However, the memories of the agony of chemotherapy and radiation were still present.

The fear of getting sick again grew day by day. Until my biggest nightmare came true during a follow-up inspection in March.

During a follow-up check in PET-CT, the doctors found a dark spot on the lungs. And in fact, I had cancer again. This time in the lungs.

I was at the end, had done so much to get better. And then this. The cancer in my bowel was gone, but now it's in my lungs.

It couldn't be! It couldn't be! I had already been healthy, had worked normally for more than a year and felt better and better.

How on earth could that be now?

And why did it hit me of all people? Why did I of all people have to go through this hell?

I didn't understand the world anymore and slowly, but surely the first depressive signs turned into a full-grown depression.

I was at the end of my rope. Emaciated and broken.

Since the tumor in the lung was still very young, the chances of getting rid of it were quite high.

At least a ray of hope in this darkness. I hoped so much that the doctors would be right, and the tumor was quick and easy to fight.

Well, I again agreed to chemotherapy, but this time it only lasted a week.

I was actually lucky, and the tumor disappeared after only one chemo.

But the fear was over helming. Fear that the doctors would find something during the follow-up check. That the tumor wasn't completely destroyed after all.

Had I finally made it, or was there another negative surprise?

The follow-up inspection in May was more than sobering. The tumor in the lung was gone. I had defeated him.

As much as I had hoped that the examination would show a complete recovery, I was disappointed.

Something was found again. This time there were large metastases in the liver.

The operation I was advised to undergo, however, I refused for the time being. I wanted to get another opinion first.

But even if I was now suffering from a full-grown depression and my self-confidence was like zero, my mind was still clear.

My decision not to trust the first doctor should still be confirmed.

After some discussions with different doctors, among them also a very well-known liver surgeon from Altötting, was certain:

No surgery! Much too dangerous!

The cancer had trapped the blood vessels to the heart and again I faced a chance of survival of less than 5%.

I suffered from shortness of breath and already had 5cm metastases.

What was I supposed to do? Have an operation, or would you rather have chemo? Neither was without it. The surgery was risky, chemo for the body actually too strenuous. My immune system was weakened, the chemo had many side effects and I was still suffering from the psychological consequences of the last two years. And it would be the third chemo in a row.
I didn't want to sit home sick again. I didn't feel like getting sick again. Self-doubt ate through my soul.
Should I really do this torment to myself again, or should I accept my fate and accept that I would die?

In the following months I was exposed to an inner struggle that almost drove me mad. I could, no, I just didn't want to make up my mind. For me, neither one nor the other alternative was a real solution. Both scared me. And to endure this fear cost me an awful lot of strength. I decided to do psychotherapy so I wouldn't go crazy. It couldn't go on like this. The fear, the desire to die and the pain were destroying my feelings. I suffered from depression and not only once did I seriously think about ending this madness and putting an end to my life.
But I couldn't wait that long either. The cancer progressed inexorably and with each passing day my chance of recovery decreased.

By the time I had finally come to my conclusion and the treatment could begin, it was already August.

Until 31.7.2018 I still worked and despite the increasing pain I decided not to let myself write sick.

My oncologist once again made it clear to me that I had to prepare myself for a difficult journey.

In August I was an outpatient at the Rosenheim Clinic for a computer-controlled biopsy. And then came the confusion. The tumor was obviously gone. No cancer cells could be detected with the biopsy. Since my oncologist wanted to be on the safe side, she sent me again for a second biopsy to Munich to the Klinikum rechts der Isar.

And there was another tumor

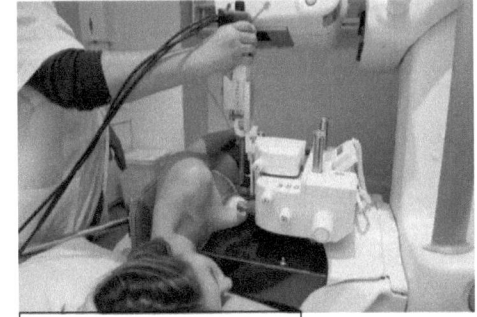

Source: Adobe Stock

detected. As it turned out, the doctors in Rosenheim had accidentally stung it and thus not removed any cancer cells.

This incident confirmed to me how important it is never to rely on a single opinion, especially for such diagnoses. Such mistakes can happen to anyone. But if we don't have it checked out, another doctor can't fix it.

For a period of eleven weeks I was given cisplatin and 5FU (both drugs that are used in combination as chemotherapy to destroy the cell walls).

The side effects were very serious. After two weeks, my voice left me, and my eyesight began to deteriorate. Arms

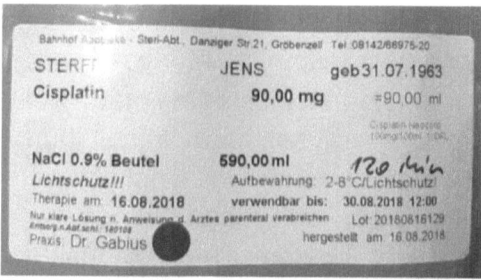

and legs were failing more and more, until I could hardly walk anymore.

I would not have been able to take care of myself without the support of friends and neighbors. I was pumped to the top with various medications, because chemotherapy could also severely damage other organs, such as the kidneys.

In addition to the physical complaints, there was the troubled psyche. Being dependent on other people just to eat something or even leave the house is one of the worst things I could imagine. I had been independent all my life, had always paid attention to be dependent on nothing and nobody and to have my life under control.

Especially the independence was very important for me after my very difficult childhood.

And then I fell ill with an illness that cost me everything that was valuable to me. My girlfriend, my independence and last but not least my independence.

I was trapped in my body, gagged by the drugs. The cancer had me under control.

Since I couldn't speak anymore, the communication was very difficult. By that time, I had almost completely lost my sight.

Since my body needed a lot of vitamins, I almost only fed on fruit and vegetables. In addition, I stuck to my soda mixture and combined my diet with CBD oil.

It was already November when the chemo was finally over. But the recovery from the side effects took time. A lot of time.

Two weeks after the end of the treatment at least my voice slowly came back, which made communication much easier.

Daily exercise in the fresh air didn't bring my legs back immediately, but my muscular strength built up again. Since good muscles in the legs are known to be an absolute prerequisite for being able to walk at all, I concentrated very strongly on my daily sports units.

Slowly I seemed to be feeling better and the follow-up check at the end of November showed that the tumor had actually shrunk by about two thirds.

The fight wasn't won yet. The tumor was still visible in the liver.

I had to move on.

And so, the radiation followed in December 2018.

I opted for stereotactic irradiation, as this only had to be used three times due to its much higher radiation dose.

This time I was treated in Rosenheim, because the hospital Rosenheim is specialized in stereotactic radiation.

I continued to suffer from severe depression. Every day was a fight. Not only the stories about people who did not survive cancer robbed me of my strength. Death had become a constant companion. I always had him before my eyes, couldn't turn my thoughts away from him.
I was in the hospital every day with other cancer patients together. Every day I saw the suffering that cancer brings. Every day began with the awareness that it might be the last. Every evening I closed my eyes and didn't know which of my many fellow patients I would see alive the next day. Or if I'd wake up again myself.

Should I just make my own decision to leave? Why wait and see if I was going to die anyway? Actually, I could put an end to my life. That'd be the end of it. I would no longer have pain, would no longer see the suffering every day - and the cancer would have won!
And that's exactly what I didn't want. My ego kept me alive. I wanted to prove that it was possible to have one's life in one's hands and win even in such a hopeless situation.

2019 - Won the fight?

On 2.1.2019 I finally went on rehab to Bayrisch Gmain. 6 weeks in the Berchtesgadener Land should help me to recover from the strains of chemo.
While my sight was finally completely back, the numbness in my legs was still there. Every step cost me an awful lot of strength.

In the course of rehab, however, I felt better and better. I refuelled, got my mental strength back and my body could recover more and more.
But despite the positive results, the final discussion with the senior physician was very sober.
She confirmed what could be read on the Internet: Metastases in the liver usually lead to death! Within the first two years after treatment, only about 5% of those affected survive.

But not with me! I had fought my way this far and had already defeated two other cancers. I also wanted to defeat the liver metastases!
Surrender wasn't an option. Not for me!

Back from rehab I was sent back to Prien at the end of February for another MRI. The result was very satisfactory: the metastases and the tumor had completely receded. MRI showed no more shadows in the liver.
But I now had a thrombus in my groin, probably caused by chemo. Right in the main vein to the lungs.

The danger of a pulmonary embolism was enormously high, so I had to spare myself accordingly in order not to risk anything.

But despite the danger of pulmonary embolism, I weighed myself in safety.

After all, the cancer was defeated. The MRI was inconspicuous.

However, when I visited my oncologist, she told me that she could not imagine that there would actually be no more metastases.

She insisted on another MRI to make sure nothing was missed in Prien.

I went into the tube again. This time in Munich, in the Klinikum rechts der Isar.

And the doctor's suspicions were confirmed: But there's something else to see!

This couldn't be happening! Which MRI was the right one?

The words of the attending only made my fear stronger. When he saw me, he greeted me with the words, "You're still alive?"

Well, that gives you hope. The doctor hadn't even expected to see me alive again. But the fact that he was convinced that I was going to die reminded me again that I was actually terminally ill.

Except for me, no one had really believed until then that I could actually defeat the cancer and survive the strains of the treatment.

In April, another MRT was ordered in Munich. The oncologist wanted to check whether the tumor in the liver was again proliferating. But this time I came back with a positive result: What can still be seen is probably only dead tumor tissue. No more cancer!

Since June I am completely healthy again.
The side effects of chemo are overcome, I can talk again, see and even my legs do their duty again.
The thrombus in the leg has also disappeared. My daily sports workload has already reached my old level.

And my psyche? This has also recovered somewhat as the healing progresses. It would be a lie to claim that I have already been completely restored psychologically. The hardships of the last few years are still deep in my bones, and every day I consciously decide not to let myself be pulled down by the memories of the last few years.
But it gets better. Every day I wake up and, contrary to doctors' predictions, start the day full of life, I become more confident. With every new day that I have been given, I am grateful for what I have.
And as hard as the years of struggle were, I'm coming out of this fight stronger than I went in.
I've learned that you can't take everything for granted and how important it is not to lose sight of the little things and be grateful for every day you wake up healthy.

Since June I have only been waiting to finally go back to work.

Because I thankfully rejected the reduced earning capacity pension that the pension insurance company offered me.
After all, life starts all over again!

When I went to the last check-up in July, my thoughts went a little crazy again. The fear of not being allowed to go to work again, or even of getting a crushing message again, was still resonating.
Fortunately, the fear has not been confirmed. My doctors were able to give me the good news that my fight against cancer had paid off. I'm healthy, my body's cancer-free. Chemotherapy and radiation left no trace in my body.
I am fully operational again and can finally go back to work.

Life can start all over again!

Genesung ↑

Krebs

What nutrition has to do with cancer

Anyone who has ever been more intensively involved with nutrition and the various nutrients knows that you can achieve a lot with the right diet.

During a normal day, our body is constantly exposed to heavy stress. Everyday products such as hair shampoo, soap or cleaning products contain substances that can be harmful to our body in large quantities.

Thus we provide completely automatically, only by our daily body care, for the fact that in our body a harmful, overacidified, milieu develops. This acidified environment is ideal for the colonisation of bacteria, for example, and cancer cells.

Here we can take a lot of countermeasures by paying attention to a healthy diet that keeps our acid-base balance in balance.

It is not necessary to switch completely to a vegan diet. But it helps me personally to keep my body in balance. Reducing the number of animal products in our diet, largely dispensing with fast food and convenience foods and preferring healthy whole meal bread instead of white flour products are, however, very good steps in the right direction.

Too much sugar, which unfortunately is standard in many foods, also damages our body and changes the environment in the intestines.

In addition, we should finally learn to resort to regional products from organic farming. All the insecticides etc.

damage our body enormously and can be responsible for cancer among other things.

A very healthy, unfortunately far too much into the background moved, food is dandelion.

Many people don't even know that we humans can eat and digest dandelions completely. It contains an incredible amount of vitamins and nutrients, such as vitamin K, which is responsible for blood clotting and bone metabolism in our body. With 100g dandelion daily a person has already covered 50 % of the vitamin C requirement. If you make a salad out of dandelion, the 100g are quickly reached.

The plant known as "rabbit food" does not only help against kidney diseases. Dandelions are a very good choice for controlling intestinal complaints or heartburn. In addition, dandelion grows almost everywhere and is therefore free of charge.

Paying attention to an alkaline diet does not heal everything, nor does it 100% prevent you from becoming ill. However, the risk of developing cancer decreases significantly. And so we also help our body to maintain or gain a healthy weight.

Sport, the right diet and taking care of my breathing have helped me to recharge my batteries and find my way back to a new life.

I already mentioned in the book that I consume various nutrients through dietary supplements and homemade drinks. In the following I have summarized the dietary supplements and the recipes for the homemade drinks for you once again.

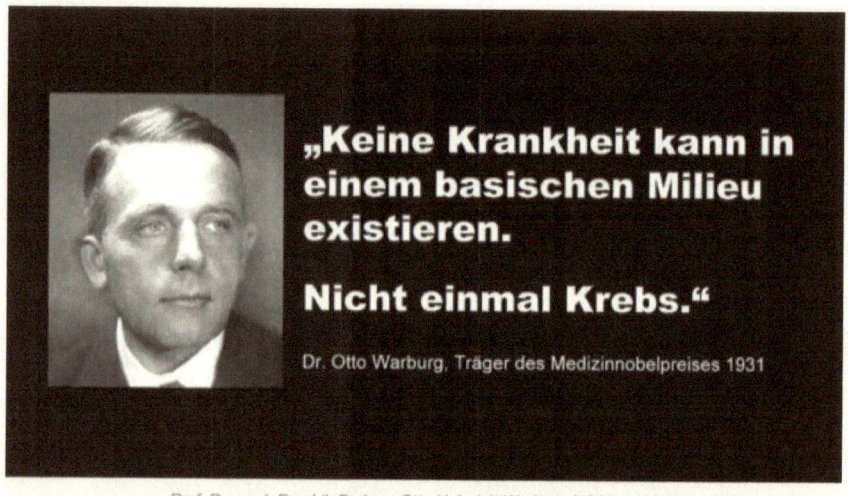

„Keine Krankheit kann in einem basischen Milieu existieren.

Nicht einmal Krebs."

Dr. Otto Warburg, Träger des Medizinnobelpreises 1931

Prof. Dr. med. Dr. phil. Dr. h. c. Otto Heinrich Warburg (1883 – 1970)

The recipes at a glance:

Magnesium chloride solution

Dissolve 100 grams of magnesium chloride in 3 litres of water (33 grams per litre) and then store in bottles (IMPORTANT: do not use plastic bottles).

Dose = one shot glass full of the prepared solution.

It's best to take it right after getting up or after coffee. Taken on an empty stomach, it is a light laxative and is excreted very quickly.

Magnesium chloride is hardly absorbed by the intestine, hence the laxative effect (which makes many people very happy). Whenever anything heals anything, it's very doubtful. Magnesium has its justification in certain complaints and real magnesium deficiency occurs. But then you should take an orally well resorbed version, i.e. magnesium glycerophosphate.

IMPORTANT: Please never buy such mixtures in the free trade, because it is not guaranteed that only the desired ingredients have been processed. The solution can be ordered from any pharmacy.

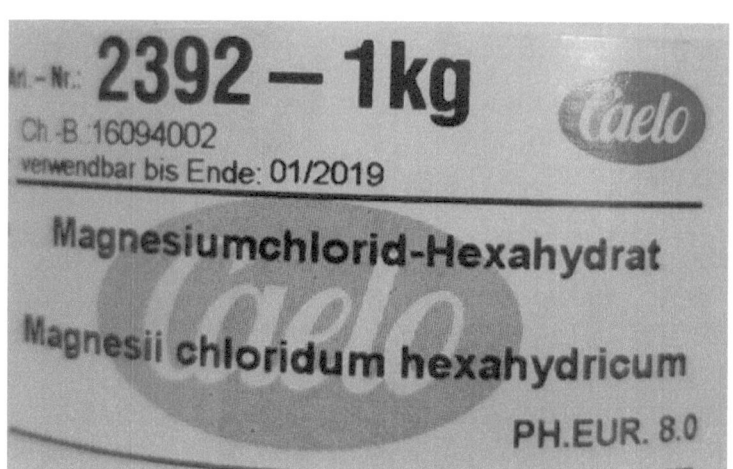

Art.-Nr.: **2392 – 1kg**
Ch.-B 16094002
verwendbar bis Ende: 01/2019

Magnesiumchlorid-Hexahydrat

Magnesii chloridum hexahydricum

PH.EUR. 8.0

This picture is a photograph of the solution I order from the pharmacy. Since I use a lot of it, I always get 1Kg. This saves shipping costs and I don't have to order so often.

Lemon cider vinegar drink

This drink is actually a true miracle cure for everyone. It strengthens the immune system (very important in chemo), helps against inflammation (also internally) and helps to recharge the electrolyte balance.
Fresh ginger is rich in vitamins B1, B2, B3 and C as well as potassium, calcium and sodium. Ginger is analgesic and anti-inflammatory.
Organic apple cider vinegar has an antibacterial effect, prevents hyperacidity and prevents heartburn.
Lemon is very rich in vitamin C and rich in antioxidants.
One liter of this drink should be consumed daily.

During the day: 1 litre of water, a squeezed organic lemon, half a grated frozen lemon with peel from the freezer, some ginger and three tablespoons of organic apple vinegar.

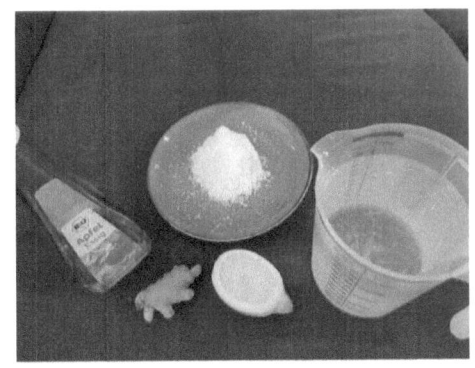

Picture source: Photography by Jens

Sodium bicarbonate solution

Sodium is taken with maple syrup because the sugar helps the cells to absorb the sodium. And sodium bicarbonate destroys the cancer cells.

Sodium powder can also be used for bathing.
3 times a week at 37 degrees.

In the evening: A glass of water (lukewarm) with 5 grams of baking soda and two teaspoons of organic maple syrup.

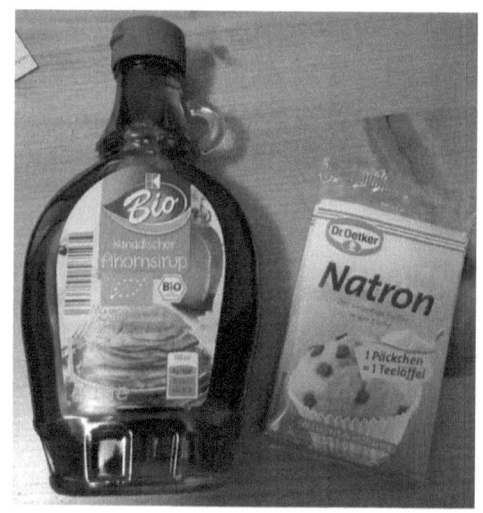

Picture source: Photography Jens Sterff

Food supplement

Since I usually eat vegan the body needs some food supplements.

For three years I have been taking the following things daily:

OPC
astaxanthin
MSM
D3
K2
zinc
vitamin B complex
Performance Probiotic
Moringa
turmeric
Magnesium - Oil
Lemon cider vinegar drink
sodium bicarbonate solution

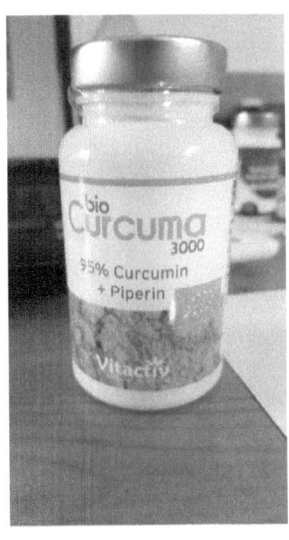

Bio-Curcuma from Vitaktiv.
Photo: Jens Sterff

Further titles of the author

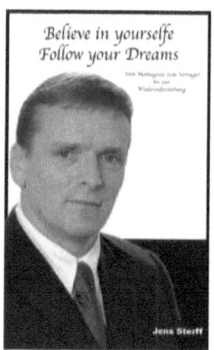

Born a twin, rejected by her mother, deported to a children's home.

My life began anything but as you would wish for a newborn baby. My parents wanted another child and were surprised with twins. There was no room for me, so I had to leave.

18 years in the children's home were the result, 18 years marked by abuse, rape, rejection. 18 years, in which my family lived only 2km away from me - and couldn't once overcome themselves to send me at least a birthday card.

The fighting spirit in me bit through. After school he trained as a restaurant specialist, then retrained as an industrial clerk. Later I studied psychology, mathematics and computer technology.

I became a member of Club Mensa - a club for highly intelligent people.

But all the intelligence, all the knowledge and my above-average education did not save me from failing again and again.

I was a typical orphan through and through. Little to no self-confidence and still became a millionaire. And failed just as fast as I had won before. I was confronted with an almost unmanageable mountain of debt of over 300,000€ and got up again.

Until I was diagnosed with cancer in 2015. Chances of survival: less than 5%.

My biography tells how little intelligence prevents us from failing. And how much a good fighting spirit helps us to get up again and win.
I want to encourage people never to give up and to use even the hardest blows of fate as an opportunity. As a chance to change, to start anew and to grow with the difficulties.

Expected publication date: April 2020